THE STRICKER METHOD

Christian Stricker

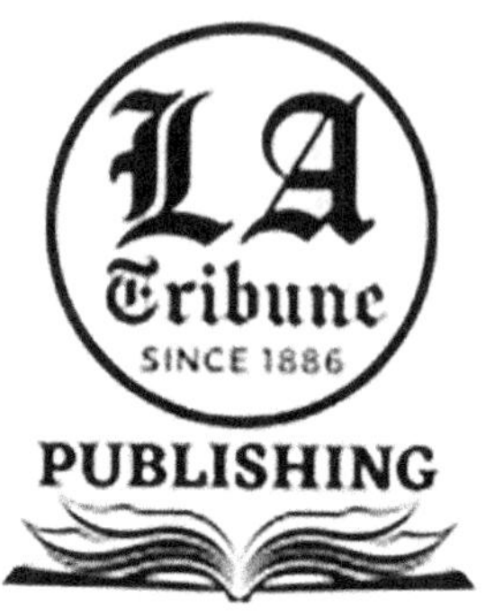

LA Tribune Publishing
205 West 300 South, Brigham City, Utah 84302

Printed in the United States of America

ISBN 979-8-8693-8490-4

Acknowledgements

I would like to acknowledge first and foremost my parents, Andy and Sue Stricker, as they raised me and provided me with the tools to pursue whatever it was that I chose and are the reason that I'm here today with the gifts that I have in regards to training, intelligence and my literary abilities.

Next, I would like to thank my great friend who is at this point, family to me, Teresa Lawrence who has continually pushed me to do something more with what I was given and get my message out into the world. She has been incredibly proactive about inspiring and motivating me to write this book, develop my business and live a life that is in line with my values and gifts.

I would like to thank all of the gym owners that I have worked for as they have given me the basis in which I could develop my training philosophy and the tools in which to test my different ideas and expose me to many different modes, methods and ways of training to find the ideal combination of effective ways to program and ways to use all of the different implements. In addition to the owners I have worked for, I would like to thank the coaches that I've had over the years, namely Burley Hawk and Kavan Woodcock, who have given me great insights into what great programming looks like from a variety of different philosophies and styles. Strength and conditioning is very much an art in addition to the science and it takes exceptional creativity to make a program safe, fun, effective and interesting.

I would also like to thank the many different training partners and clients that I have had over the years as they have exposed me to different ideas and ways of thinking, given me inspiration for many different ideas and forced me to get creative with how I create my different training programs to most effectively serve them.

About the Author

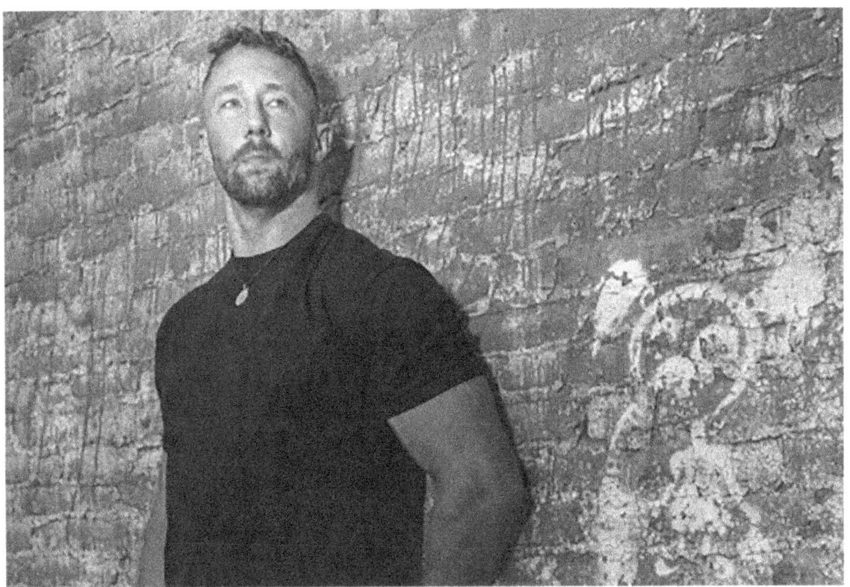

Ever since I was a child, I have always been interested in what I could do with my body. Whether it was testing my strength attempting to lift the largest rock or log down at the creek at my childhood home, jumping from our roof to our trampoline and then from that one to our second one with however many flips and spins I could complete before landing or testing my speed, agility, strategy and tactics in games of paintball. Once I found strength training due in part to my high school friend Kurt Sorensen, it was a near limitless and unending way to see what was possible both physically and intellectually as getting stronger is as much of an intellectual pursuit as it is physical in that you need to get smarter about training and recovery to get stronger. The stronger you get, the harder it is to get stronger and so the smarter and more knowledgeable you must become to continue making progress. I took it upon myself to learn formally from my time completing my Bachelor's Degree in Exercise and Sport Science from Oregon State University (where I learned almost nothing about how to program for strength training but learned about how the body worked). Most of my education in making myself stronger and teaching others, came from YouTube University. I also found various written resources available online from the people training some of the strongest people in the world such as Dave Tate of Elite FTS, Louie Simmons at Westside Barbell, Travis Mash at Mash Elite and Greg Everett at Catalyst Athletics as well as many others. After having some success with my own training in how it made me feel, my physical/athletic performance and in the aesthetic improvements it afforded me, training other people to experience the same benefits was the next natural progression. This would happen informally just imparting the knowledge I had gained to my training partners then in more formal settings such as coaching CrossFit in the various different gyms I worked at throughout Oregon. I coached CrossFit for many years and at this point, the number of people that I have coached to improve their lives through physical training is likely in the thousands. CrossFit was a great introduction to all of the different avenues, methods and implements you can use in training, as there are multitudes. It is probably the best program to find out what kind of training you most resonate with as it utilizes them all, aerobic, strength, power, speed, stamina, etc. (agility to a small degree) and gives you exposure to almost all of the different implements you may use in your training career. I have trained and programmed many people to be at their strongest, fittest and most in shape selves. To their first 400 lbs. squat, their first 500+ lbs. deadlift and their first 300+ lbs. bench press, some of the biggest milestones a person will hit in their strength-training career. I have coached a couple of children to be as strong as or stronger than grown men.

Mighty Mission

The purpose of this book is to give you the framework for building the highest functioning body that you are capable of building with what you were genetically endowed with. It incorporates several different types of training modalities because each thing conveys different benefits to you when you regularly perform that type of exercise and contributes to your life and performance as a whole. The focus isn't just on a particular aspect of fitness/ training as everything works together to produce a high performance body that will not only improve your physical capabilities but your mental and spiritual as well as you will be enhancing the vessel in which you interact with the world. My mission is to help people develop their body and mind in a way that instills confidence and capability in an aesthetically attractive package.

Table of Contents

Introduction

When I was in high school, I was a tiny human being, so small in fact that my friends decided to call me a little bitch (partly my stature and partly my attitude of being a stubborn pain in the ass ha-ha). I weighed 98 lbs. my freshman year and to the envy of my teammates, I was able to eat whatever I wanted during wrestling season without worrying about not making weight for the lightest weight class in wrestling. While this was great for my nutrition and diet, it absolutely sucked for most other things, namely my confidence and probably my less-than-stellar results with women at the time. I was damn good at things that required skill and finesse but not so much with things that required brute strength and physicality. It was at some point during my time in high school that I was introduced to the weight room, mostly during PE, and for getting ready for football and to put on a size. The things I did were extremely basic and pretty much what you might see in a Muscle and Fitness magazine, there was no real instruction on technique and how to use your body correctly, most of the stuff I did was with dumbbells. I was somewhat interested in it and put forth more effort into it than I did into our mile run challenges (which I walked). I did not start getting really into training until after high school, when I learned that I could make my own set of Olympic rings out of warmed-up PVC pipe wrapped around a coffee can and climbing rope, which actually ended up being incredibly sturdy. I had wanted to do an iron cross and started training the things that I thought would get me there starting with chin-ups, dips, muscle ups, and cross flies starting in plank position. From there, through some of the different forums I would read about training in, I was exposed to training with the barbell. Mostly in terms of deadlifting, squatting, rows, bench pressing and overhead pressing but some other random accessory-type movements sprinkled in there as well. My form was probably atrocious and I really had no clue what good form was or why you should use it but I enjoyed lifting with whatever technique I was using and managed to not hurt myself so things were not bad.

After a few months of training like this, I had heard about something called CrossFit from one of my Friends Kurt. I quickly became obsessed with that because it fulfilled many of my favorite things about training. I loved the challenge of not knowing what I was going to be getting myself into each workout and that it never got any easier because you just got better. It was always interesting and engaging.

I trained for CrossFit for many years, competing in it and coaching it, learning everything I could about the various aspects of training from it such as strength, bodybuilding, conditioning, etc. In addition to learning how to train each aspect, I was also introduced to and learned how to effectively and efficiently use nearly all of the various implements that one would use for strength and conditioning. (Aside from the community of people that you are introduced to and bond with, these are probably the most beneficial benefits of learning and training CrossFit. Learning how to develop all of these, different qualities and how to use all of the different implements as they are all utilized at one point or another if you participate long enough with enough different gyms as I did).

After a few years of coaching and participating in CrossFit, it was really time to learn and graduate to the next tier of training, conjugate style strength training. While CrossFit was, a great introduction to how to combine a certain few movements in as many different combinations as possible, conjugate style lifting (which is different from Westside barbell's version of conjugate) was the way to vary each type of movement. It would allow for a nearly infinite number of combinations of varying not only what exercises you do but also the way you do each one and with what implement you do it with.

While my time at OSU was great when it came to meeting people, the amount of actual usable knowledge in terms of strength training was limited but thankfully, I love learning, and once I find something

That I am fascinated with. I will incessantly seek out knowledge in that area until I am satisfied and know it thoroughly enough to be proficient in it.

In fact, there was one year where I made it a point to read a book a week, 52 books in all throughout the year, partly because I had heard about the mixing and melding of knowledge that happens when you read and learn about a breadth of topics all at once. In addition, partly because I wanted to see

If I could do it. The brain is fascinating in the way it forms what seem to be random connections (which depending on what you believe, may not actually be as random as it would appear) and I'd say that learning about the brain and the way people think definitely competes with training for my primary interest. One of my favorite disciplines within the field is called Evolutionary Psychology, which posits that the mind is an organ made of modules that essentially govern your consciousness and exist to solve different problems in our collective evolutionary past, present and future.

Throughout this period, I learned from a variety of sources. Many of the things that I learned were from Louie Simmons who was preaching methods that would take decades to be confirmed by exercise scientists. They say that bro science is the science that predates university science (kind of, as if science fiction precludes science fact, maybe one causes the other to be manifested, who knows?). This is something that I have continued to do to this day, although it's much harder to come by useful, high-quality, applicable and new information at this point since I have consumed so much from so many extremely well-versed and intelligent people.

One of my great friends who we will call Your Trueness, challenged me to write this and is one of my primary inspirations for doing so as she has always believed in me and what I'm capable of even if I didn't myself. She was the one who came up with this concept of Inner Viking, The iron Will, sense of adventure, courage to explore, conquer, shape the world as they saw fit and indomitable spirit of the people who have had some of the greatest impact on the world of humankind that the world has ever seen.

As I am writing this, I think about how incredible it is to go from someone that my friends referred to as "Little Bitch", or someone who other men had no second thoughts about putting their hands on my girlfriend. Even those who did not even have to cut weight to make the lightest weight class in all of high school wrestling. To become someone who is respected by professional athletes, men in the special forces and some of the highest performing human beings on the planet and whom professional athletes and their family have personally introduced themselves to because they found out about through social media.

It is insane what can happen if you just stick to something and continue to push the boundaries of what you thought possible. This is why I love training others since I have seen just how profound not only the outer changes can be and how it affects your interactions with every other person you communicate with but also the inner changes in how much more confident you become. What you believe is possible for yourself and how much better you feel physically, mentally, emotionally and spiritually. Becoming stronger and fitter improves every aspect of your life, directly or indirectly. It makes you smarter, more confident, more capable, and more resilient, helps you make more money, puts you in a better mood and mental state, helps you look your best and even helps you meet great, successful, genuinely awesome people and who knows, could even help you find the love of your life.

CHAPTER 1

Full Spectrum Training for Life and Sport

The main philosophy behind the ideas within this vessel of knowledge is a guide to optimal performance as the human machine that you are. Each aspect of training confers certain benefits and by performing that type of training regularly, you will start to realize those benefits. This is meant to address all of the fundamentals of training that will prepare you for more specific work down the road if you choose to play a sport or practice martial arts. It is for optimal performance as a human and why each aspect is important so you know you're not just doing something just to do it and can manipulate how and when you do something to achieve particular goals or figure out what aspect may be holding you back from achieving what you want to achieve.

1. Aerobic Fitness and General Physical Preparedness (GPP)

   - Increases your body's ability to tolerate higher workloads in strength training so you can continue to make progress.

     o Sometimes a lack of aerobic fitness and GPP can hold back your strength training due to being unable to recover from the stresses of performing the increasingly higher amounts of training volume that are necessary to make progress in your lifting.

   - Increases your stress tolerance.

     o Performing aerobic exercise increases your ability to tolerate stress in other areas of your life in a real, physiological way. Your body is making actual Physiological adaptations, not just altering your psychological perception of stressors, that allow you to deal with stress easier than it would if you were not in proper aerobic condition. This works in addition to the Subjectively perceived, psychological stress reduction that comes along with this type of training.

     o Many people who are in high-stress careers or environments who perform some sort of aerobic training or are in great aerobic shape are able to last much longer and avoid burnout better than their peers who avoid such training. It allows you to perform at a higher level and for longer than you otherwise would. This is true among members of the military, executives in business, business owners and other similarly stressful lines of work.

- It increases your longevity and prevents disease.
  - Aerobic exercise is one of the few things that has been shown to help you live a longer, more capable life. This is for a variety of factors including disease prevention from many different forms of cancer and most lifestyle-related Diseases as these diseases often originate from a lack of activity and stagnation within the body and its cells of some sort. It increases your ability to efficiently eliminate toxins and waste which are culprits to disease.
- Increases intra-workout efficiency and recovery.
  - being able to recover quickly between heavy and difficult sets of strength and hypertrophy work is largely related to your aerobic conditioning, aerobic capacity and aerobic power. Being in proper aerobic shape helps, you to recover quicker than if you were out of shape allowing you to get through your planned workouts quicker than if you were Deconditioned.

- Increases inter-workout recovery.
  - being in great, aerobic shape means that your body almost certainly has a well-developed vascular network that distributes nutrient and oxygen-rich blood to all areas of the body efficiently and effectively. Since your circulatory system delivers the nutrients that repair your body through your blood, blood flow is key when it comes to repairing and recovering fatigued and/or damaged tissues and promoting healing to areas of the body that have been damaged and fatigued through training. Having a well-developed circulatory system and performing exercise that increases circulation throughout the body promotes healing and recovery.
- being well conditioned allows you to demonstrate your strength and other athletic qualities for longer and with greater quality.
  - The better your conditioning is, the longer you can demonstrate your strength and power. This also applies to your coordination as performing skills under extreme fatigue is much more difficult than when performing them when you are still fresh. This is most applicable to sport and combat where being able to perform at a high level

when you are under fatigue and the stakes are high is critical and could be the difference between winning and losing or life and death.

- You will be able to think clearer, quicker, and better when you are aerobically fit and performing exercise that promotes blood flow.

  - Exercise increases and improves circulation throughout the body, this includes the brain. The more blood that gets to the brain, the more nutrients and oxygen it has to perform its physiological processes and the cognitive work that it does. Whether it was taking long walks or bike rides through the city or performing more rigorous exercises, many of the world's most famous geniuses such as Benjamin Franklin and Nikola Tesla, were known to have also been avid exercisers in some form.

  - Aerobic exercise is also known to increase a compound called BDNF that is in part responsible for the growth of new neurons and in maintaining neuroplasticity. This protein is important for forming new connections between your neurons, for learning and for protecting your currently neurological network. Essentially, aerobic training makes you smarter, able to learn more efficiently and more resistant to cognitive decline and diseases related to the brain such as Alzheimer's and Dementia.

- It reduces your need for sleep and helps you sleep deeper. While this is somewhat anecdotal, it seems to be consistent amongst all that I have talked to. When you start regularly performing aerobic exercise and start to get into better condition, you start to need less sleep to feel rested. It helps you to sleep deeper and to require less sleep to recuperate.

How

The easiest way to implement aerobic exercise is to just start walking. It is THAT easy. As little as 20 minutes a day is enough to greatly mitigate your risk of many lifestyle-related diseases and improve, you are conditioning if you are not currently doing anything. Eventually, you want to work up to around 10000 steps a day throughout the day. This is more in line with the daily activity that our ancestors performed and what our bodies evolved to do and leads to optimal health and body composition as well as the whole host of benefits that we discussed earlier. Since you are increasing the blood flow to the brain and promoting BDNF production, it is a great time to contemplate, listen to and learn from an audiobook or podcast or make it social with a friend or group of friends. Some very successful entrepreneurs and businesses have walking meetings, as the movement tends to increase creative thinking and problem solving.

In addition to just walking, it's important to perform low-intensity steady-state (LISS) cardio as it makes changes to your heart that allow it to work less hard during exercise and daily living, increasing its efficiency. The low-intensity nature of this method allows you to accumulate some significant time training without increasing the stress hormones that your body tends to produce with higher-intensity methods and can be more beneficial for your body composition because of this. Since it is typically performed at a higher intensity than a walk, it is better for increasing BDNF production. You want to aim to do something aerobic (running, rowing, biking, ski erg, dragging a light sled, etc.) at a pace that is moderately difficult for 30 minutes most days of the week.

Low(er) intensity intervals are the next step in the hierarchy of aerobic exercise. Once you've been performing the above for several weeks and have improved your conditioning to the point where the above activities are fairly easy, it's time to start playing around with low-intensity intervals as they more closely resemble the type of exertion that you'd be experiencing in sports and life. These are performed at a pace that is faster than the pace you would use for low-intensity steady state work but not quite high enough to be exceptionally challenging. These types of intervals can be performed 2-3 times a week for 8-12 rounds of a minute of work followed by a minute of active rest/recovery or 8-12 rounds at a slightly faster pace for 15 seconds of work and 60 seconds of active recovery.

High-intensity intervals are one of the most effective ways to increase your conditioning and improve your body composition but they can also be extremely fatiguing and only need to be performed 1-2 times a week to get their benefits. If you perform them too much, they will lose effectiveness, as your body will be under too much stress to recover from them. This can lead to burnout, unwanted weight gain, and possible injury. When performed in the right dosage, they are great and very effective in improving your health, body composition, and cognitive abilities. Some of the best intervals are 5-15 seconds at a pace you can go all out for the work period followed by 1-2 minutes active rest depending on how hard you were working. If you are having a tough time recovering, give yourself a bit longer break so you can maximize the intensity of each set. Think about taking the minimum break that you need to be able to give the same effort as the previous interval but no longer.

CHAPTER 2

Strength Training

Strength is your ability to overcome or resist particular forces (this applies to more than just physical) and impart your will onto the environment, others, and in regards to moving your body. Along with aerobic training, strength is one of the most fundamental physical capacities of the body. It essentially governs how well you will be able to develop almost any other athletic quality, although, strength and hypertrophy go nearly hand in hand as they each require the other for optimal development. Strength is how much force you can create in a given range of motion and movement pattern, whether it's being able to carry all the bags of groceries from your car to the house in one trip, pushing yourself up off the ground, pulling yourself up onto a ledge or playfully throwing your girlfriend over your shoulder to transport her around. These are all different ranges and demonstrations of strength.

Strength is a continuum and ranges from something as simple as just being able to crawl to flying through a ninja warrior obstacle course as fast as possible to deadlifting over 1000 pounds. Each of these activities requires a different level and type of strength and represents different investments of time, dedication, and attention to training this particular quality, which happens to be one of the most trainable physical characteristics along with aerobic capacity. Strength gives you options in regards to moving your own body, other things or people, and being able to manipulate your environment on your own. Someone who is weaker may only be able to crawl around to move from one place to another but someone who is strong has the option to crawl, walk, jog, sprint, jump, or do all of the above while carrying someone or an object that weighs several hundred pounds. They have their choice in how they want to move and are not limited by their physical condition in how they choose to move.

Due to having more options with how to move your body and the things around you, you become a more useful person. Not that you're some sort of tool but that in the event that you or someone else needs something done or needs help, especially in an emergency, you won't be limited by your physical capacity and you won't have to rely on outside tools or help to accomplish the things you're trying to do. This could range from being able to lift your groceries onto the counter to being able to carry a couch or mattress up several flights of stairs by yourself. If you are not strong enough to do these things, you will have to rely on outside help to get the jobs done. Having greater strength gives you greater physical independence.

Being strong makes, you tougher, more resilient and durable in all respects and if you get strong enough, it can serve as a conflict deterrent for those around you as well. In interviews with sex offenders and child traffickers, when asked about how they would choose their victims and what would deter them from doing so, they state that they would look at the dad or male figure around the child. If the dad appeared weak and inattentive, like they would not notice or be able to do anything about it if they did, the predator would be much more likely to kidnap the child. If the male appeared formidable, as if they could do something about it, they would be much less likely to attempt to kidnap the child. Simply being bigger, stronger, and more imposing helps you to avoid conflict in the first place. When you are smaller and weaker, some people tend to think they can do what they want and treat you how they like, which is poorly in some cases. When you are big, strong, physically fit, and imposing, people in most cases will give you a certain basic level of respect and treat you with such. In addition to deterring other people from engaging in conflict with you or those around you, your body is simply strong and resilient enough to withstand more outside force being imparted on it such as falling down, getting in an accident, being hit, etc. Every structure in your body gets stronger when you start strength training, the bones, the ligaments, the tendons, and of course, the muscles all adapt to the stress that you are putting on them by getting stronger, and as long as this process is gradual and the dose of training is in the right amount, the structures will not break in the process. This process is called hormesis, the application of some sort of stressor that when applied in an optimal amount, will trigger a rebuilding response in the body that makes it stronger than it was prior to the stress and will make it more resilient to it the next time it encounters it. If the stressor is not enough, the body will remain the same, as the adaptation threshold was not reached, if too much is applied, then the structure may break causing an injury.

In athletics, strength is what some would call the "Mother quality" from which all other qualities are derived. The stronger you are, the more powerful you can become as power is force applied over a period. To increase power, you can increase the force or decrease the amount of time it takes to apply that force/increase the speed at which it is applied. With strength being one of the most trainable qualities there is and speed being one of the least trainable, it makes sense to put most of your training efforts into getting stronger. A person's max strength can also improve their single set repetitions to failure at lighter weights as well (aerobic capacity coming into play more with longer single set and multiset durations). If one person can squat 500 pounds, they will be able to do more reps at 250 pounds than someone whose max is 300 pounds.

When you are strong, nearly everything is easier. This is not just a physical phenomenon but also mentally as almost everything seems easier when you are regularly strength training and pushing your limits as it is always challenging. If you're doing things right, it never gets easier, you just get stronger and thus have to put out the same amount of effort each time albeit with more resistance. You get so accustomed to putting out such a high degree of effort that those things that do not take that much effort seem a hell of a lot easier. This makes daily life less fatiguing and helps you deal with the stresses of it much better. Having discussed this topic with several high-performing executives, business owners, and people in highly stressful lines of work such as the military and some trades, this along with aerobic training or martial arts of some sort is what allows many high achievers to continue achieving at high levels past the point where their peers would have burned out. It allows you to avoid and prevents burnout.

How

Strength is best developed in conjunction with building muscle as the amount of muscle you have affects how strong you can ultimately become. Building muscle at the same time as you build strength will allow you to get stronger for longer than if you just purely worked on developing strength. Thankfully, many of the methods that are used to build strength will also help you to build the accompanying muscle along with it, although this is not always the case especially when it comes to methods that primarily train the neurological aspect of strength. The neurological aspect is essentially the strength of the signal that your body sends to your muscles to contract in a certain pattern, for instance, a deadlift.

This is largely developed by regularly and consistently performing the motion and with an intensity that is great enough to cause the body to adapt and compensate to a higher level. Therefore, you need muscle to have the raw materials to produce strength and you need the neurological drive to be able to fully utilize the amount of muscle you have during a given movement.

In the most basic terms, the closer to failure that you take a given set, the better it will be for building muscle. One technique you can use to gauge this is to take the set to the point where your rep speed involuntarily slows down the most while still being able to complete the set. Building muscle can be done with anywhere between 4-30 reps as long as the set is done until just before failure. Depending on your goals, you can perform the sets in a way that will build either strength or endurance by doing your hypertrophy with lower reps (4-10) or endurance (10+ reps). Working up to your one rep max will be great in terms of building strength but will not build much muscle unless you do the right assistance work afterwards. Assistance and accessory work is used to build up both muscular deficiencies and deficiencies in strength through a certain range of motion that is currently weak relative to the rest. In terms of strengthening a specific range of motion for a movement, you would want to choose an assistance lift that is similar to the one you are trying to build. As an example, if you are weak through the middle range of motion on a deadlift, the mid-shin to the mid-thigh, you could do Romanian deadlifts or RDLs, a movement that specifically works that range of motion and helps you to improve your strength through it. In addition to RDLs, you could also do exercises that build the muscles in the low back, glutes and hamstrings, which are highly active throughout that range of motion. These could include reverse hyperactive, back raises; machine or band leg curls of all types and GHD raises or inverse curls, personal favorites of mine.

When it comes to building strength, you will want to stay within the 1-6 rep range and for most people who are not concerned with the absolute most weight they can lift for some sort of sport or event, you will want to stay within the 3-6 rep range, as this will help you build both strength and muscle. You can do singles and doubles to test out how you are progressing on your lifts but ultimately, you will be better served by developing both your strength and your aesthetics. In terms of sets, you'll want to do 3-6 sets, working up to the heaviest weight that you're capable of doing with good technique for the target number of reps for that day and continually trying to improve on that over time.

General Workout Structure

In short, you choose the primary movement that you want to get better at or something that is very similar to it. For instance, if you want to get stronger at the squat and anything else that the squat transfers to, you could start your workout by working up to a three rep max squat, box squat or pin squat. After you hit your top set on the squat, you can do a back off set or two for higher reps with less weight or move immediately into your assistance work.

Your first assistance exercise would be something that resembles a squat or specifically builds the squat. This could be a good morning if your back strength is what limits you in the squat, a belt squat or unilateral leg strengthening exercise such as a lunge if your legs are the limiter or single leg deadlift or hip extension if your hips are the limiters.

Next you would choose something that builds up muscularly deficient areas that is low risk and is a mostly "isolation" type exercise such as a GH raise, inverse curl, machine leg curl, back extension or reverse hyper. Next, you could do another exercise in a similar vein; aiming to get at least one low back strengthening isolation type exercise each lower body day. Finally, rounding out the training session with some abdominal or oblique train-ing exercises will help you ensure that your torso is stay-ing strong and resilient.

In terms of what an upper body workout might look like, let us say you are trying to build your bench press and your sticking point is through the middle of the move-ment. You also have somewhat underdeveloped triceps relative to the rest of your musculature and relative to other people who have a bigger bench press than you do. This combination of being weak through the mid-dle of the movement where the triceps are highly active and having somewhat smaller triceps points towards your triceps being the weak point. To really hammer this weakness, we would do a primary bench press variation that is an analog of the standard bench press such as a regular bench, paused bench or pin bench press.

Then as a secondary assistance lift, something that resembles the main movement but builds your specific weak point, we could choose a close grip bench press since it develops that specific range of motion and puts extra emphasis on the triceps.

Then, as the third movement, we would do a dumb-bell Tate press since this works the triceps through this specific range of motion. And to finish out, we would hit either another triceps accessory or start in on a row vari-ation to keep the upper body balanced and the shoul-ders healthy and finish out the workout with a rear delt/external rotation developing exercise to again, keep the shoulders healthy and prevent injury to the rear delts from having overdeveloped internal rotators and under-developed external rotators.

If you have a very glaring weakness, you can adjust this structure to add another assistance/accessory exercise to accommodate for that. It is important to ensure that you are getting adequate volume in each week for the particular weakness you are aiming to build while not completely neglecting things you are already strong at.

General Weekly Schedule and Small Training Block Schedule

Each week, you will want to have a plan for what you are going to work on. There are different aspects of strength that all interact with each other to produce your strongest self and it is important to touch on each of these aspects each week and periodically rotate the focus depending on your strengths and weaknesses at the time.

The following weekly structure allows you to train hard consistently as you are not over emphasizing any particular aspect for too long. It is all right to emphasize specific aspects for shorter periods to really build up a weakness but continually hammering the same thing repeatedly can lead to burnout and injury.

When it comes to creating your training block, (which is about a 4 week period of time where you focus on a specific aspect of strength training for that time period), you'll want to choose what your biggest weaknesses for both your upper body and lower body are and focus your program on developing those with your targeted assistance and accessory exercises.

If your goal is to get as strong as possible and as quickly as possible, you will want to avoid just doing general strength programs. If you do a general program, you might get stronger but not at the rate in which you would if, you formulated your program to address your specific weaknesses. When you target your specific weaknesses you're also building up the areas that are most susceptible to injury as it's not the strong parts of your body that get injured, it's the weak parts. The saying, "Weak things break." is very accurate in this context.

Sample Weekly Structure *the following is the structure for the main movement of the day. The number is the number of reps you will be performing for your top set of the day. For speed days, you will use Prilepin's chart to determine the number of sets and reps per set you will be performing for that day.

Day 1 - Heavy Lower Body with heavy, lower rep assistance/accessories

Block 1) W1 - Heavy 6, W2 - Heavy 4, W3 - Deload Speed Work, W4 - Heavy 2 Block 2) W1 - Heavy 5, W2 - Heavy 3, W3 - Deload Speed Work, W4 - Heavy 1

Day 2 - Heavy Upper Body with heavier, lower rep assistance/accessories

Block 1) W1 - Heavy 6, W2 - Heavy 4, W3 - Deload Speed Work, W4 - Heavy 2 Block 2) W1 - Heavy 5, W2 - Heavy 3, W3 - Deload Speed Work, W4 - Heavy 1

Day 3 - Rest or Low Impact Aerobics Training/GPP

Day 4 - Rep/Speed/Explosive Lower Body with lighter, higher rep assistance/accessories Block 1) Speed Wave - W1 - 70%, W2 - 75%, W3 - Deload Speed Work, W4 - 80%

Block 2) Explosive Wave - W1 - 50%, W2 - 55%, W3 - Deload Speed Work, W4 - 60% Alternative Block 2) Rep Wave - W1 - AMRep at 70%, W2 - AMRep at 75%, W3 - Deload Speed Work, W4 - AMRep at 80%

Day 5 - Rep/Speed/Explosive Upper Body with lighter, higher rep assistance/accessories Block 1) Speed Wave - W1 - 70%, W2 - 75%, W3 - Deload Speed Work, W4 - 80% Block 2) Explosive Wave - W1 - 50%, W2 - 55%, W3 - Deload Speed Work, W4 - 60% Alternative Block 2) Rep Wave - W1 - AMRep at 70%, W2 - AMRep at 75%, W3 - Deload Speed Work, W4 - AMRep at 80%

Day 6 - Extra Small/Isolation Accessories and Aerobic Training/GPP

Day 7 - Rest Day and/or Easy Yoga/Mobility optional easy hike or walk

CHAPTER 3

Muscle Building/Hypertrophy - The Governor of Strength

While it is possible to get damn strong without putting on a lot of muscle due to the neurological adaptations that occur with repeated practice of particular movement patterns, ultimately, you will be limited by the amount of muscle mass you have.

Part of strength training is becoming more efficient at utilizing the muscle that you have to accomplish the tasks that you give your body. This means that you are essentially teaching your nervous system to direct more of your muscle mass and neurological drive towards the goal movement and improving the neurological drive that is sent to those muscles.

When put into numerical terms which might paint a more understandable picture, this would mean that the first time you do a movement you might use 50% of the total muscle mass you have available to use for that movement. Then the next time, you might use 52% because your body has adapted to the prior training session (these are figurative, not actual numbers).

Supposedly, it is not possible to achieve 100% muscle activation voluntarily but this is one way that your strength increases without increasing your body weight or muscle mass. Once you reach a point where your body has figured out how to use, as much of your available muscle as it can voluntarily, the only way to get stronger is to build more muscle. This is why it is important to start using methods to build as much muscle as you can while concurrently building your strength, so that you can avoid the stagnation that will likely occur once you have learned how to utilize all the muscle you have.

In addition to the performance benefits that you gain from building muscle, you will also start to build a body that you are proud of aesthetically. This will translate into greater confidence in yourself and in your attractiveness to potential partners as muscle is an indicator of health, hard work and dedication, all attractive qualities.

When you build muscle utilizing bodybuilding/hypertrophy methods, techniques, exercises and movements, that muscle will also be usable for other movements otherwise the whole field of strength and conditioning would be a waste as what you do in the weight room would only translate into the weight room and not onto the field, court, track, mat, etc. There can be differences in which direction the muscle fibers align but overall, when you build muscle, it will be usable in movements that utilize the joints that the muscle moves. Sometimes, what happens is that you may not be immediately able to utilize the new muscle until you start practicing the movement you want it to transfer to.

You can think about it like this. If you do a 6-month training block dedicated to building strength and muscle in the legs utilizing squats and various assistance lifts and you want it to transfer to something outside of the weight room like sprints, the first time you do sprints, (in this instance, let's say that you don't do them concurrently during your squat training block) after your squat training block, you may only be marginally faster or possibly not faster at all.

Then, the next time you do them, likely after several days of rest/recovery and your body and nervous system have had the chance to consolidate the stimulus from the training/activity; you will likely be significantly faster than you were before the training block (these timelines are for instance, it could take longer before you realize the results of the program). Each time you do them, you will likely see improvements until your body has figured out how to use all of the muscle and strength you have built. This is assuming that you chose the right exercises, at the right intensities and developed the right muscle groups that contribute the most to sprinting and optimally develop your specific weaknesses related to sprinting.

Now that you know why you need to start focusing on building muscle early on, let us talk about how you do that. You can use a variety of different intensities to build muscle as long as you make the set appropriately challenging. This refers to the percentage of your one RM that a given weight is and not necessarily, how difficult a set "feels" although these things can be closely tied together. Higher intensity = more weight relative to your one rep max, lower intensity = less weight relative to your one RM. You can do a variety of set and rep ranges to build muscle as long as you do enough volume each week.

Usually, this ends up being 2-5 sets of 3-15 reps done at a tempo that is controlled during the lowering portion of the lift resulting in a 3-4 second time range (the eccentric), possibly paused for anywhere between just coming to a complete stop instantaneously up to 5 or more seconds at the point where the most stretch is exhibited in the muscle that you're targeting, then coming up fast.

To maximize hypertrophy, you may want to avoid coming all the way to a full lockout and losing tension in the target muscles opting to spend most of the time during the set moving through the range of motion where there is the most stretch in the target muscle or muscle group (the bottom to middle portion of the squat, for instance). In terms of building strength, since there is a neurological component to it, it's optimal to at least occasionally practice the movements through the fullest range of motion that you're able to, especially if the activities that you do and the sports that you play utilize those ranges of motion. To truly get the most hypertrophy out of a given set, you need to take that set as close to failure as possible without failing.

A good way to gauge this is to go until the point where you have the largest involuntary drop off in the velocity of your reps as you can while still being able to complete them. The greater the involuntary drop-off in rep velocity by the end of a set while still being able to complete the reps, the greater the muscle-building stimulus will be. You can do forced reps where another person or contraption helps you to complete a rep you otherwise wouldn't have been able to but this level of difficulty is typically unnecessary for most people unless they have a significant amount of training experience and have not been making progress with standard methods.

Another advanced method is to do drop sets where when you are unable to complete any more reps with a particular weight, you rack that weight and immediately start doing reps with a lighter weight that you are still able to do. Again, this advanced method is unnecessary unless you are not making progress from methods that are more basic and everything else in your life is on point including your stress levels, sleep, and diet. These are the first things to correct if you're not making gains, then, once those aspects are optimized, it's time to start to look into modifying your approach to training and muscle building.

A more recent finding in some circles is that the hypertrophy stimulus of an exercise is greatest when you primarily focus on and perform movements mostly in the range of motion where the muscle you're training is in the most stretched position such as the bottom of the bench press (especially with dumbbells) or squat. I can attest to this as the sorest that I get is when performing slow eccentric paused squats where you only come up a quarter to halfway.

Over time, you will want to make sure that you are always trying to do things a bit better in some way. This could be in the form of doing more reps at a certain weight, or more weight for a given number of reps. Being able to control a movement better, intentionally utilizing a slower tempo, or implementing paused reps at a particular weight during a set number of reps. (extends your time under tension), And moving a weight faster during the concentric portion of the lift, using a tougher implement or variation of the movement such as doing a front squat instead of a back squat, pretty much anything that makes what you're doing more difficult. If you always do something the same way, with the same weight, you're either not going to get any better or you're going to get better at a significantly slower rate than if you were trying to improve in some way each time you do something.

Building Muscle in an Evolutionarily Attractive Way

While building muscle for performance, strength and symmetry should be your primary goal, as you will most likely end up developing an attractive physique along the way, you can direct the muscle building process in a way that maximizes your attractiveness to the opposite sex based on principles of evolutionary psychology. These principles happen to be different for men and women so your focal points will be different based on whom you want to attract but there is a surprising amount of congruence in what is considered aesthetically attractive for each sex.

Men

For men, building the body of a warrior is ideal. The underlying characteristics conveyed in this body type or more body manifestation, if you will, are physical indicators of status, (indicated by posture influenced by serotonin, strength in certain areas namely the back and spine), dominance, and competence conveyed through demonstrations of strength and essentially a top-heavy V-shaped torso with a big, broad chest and shoulders, big traps and a big, strong upper back. This is a lean physique with broad shoulders; a big, full chest; a big, strong upper back that tapers down to a narrow waist and hips; proportionately big, athletic glutes, and strong, lean but not necessarily big legs. You want to get as close to a 1.62+:1 shoulder-to-hip width ratio by building a big, full chest, bowling ball delts, a lean midsection and the appearance of narrow hips as these bodily characteristics have been shown in many studies and observations to be the most universally attractive physical qualities in males.

Women do not prefer dad bods. It is unwise to take seriously people claiming this to be true and if someone does claim this, look at whom they actually date (or more accurately, whom they have short term relationships with or lust after). Typically, women who actively choose men for this particular body type or claim they are attracted to it do so because they have a worry that a more physically attractive partner may not stay with them. Whether or not this belief is founded or unfounded is irrelevant and not within the scope of this book. While as a gender, men tend to find many different female forms attractive, the same is not true with women, as there tends to be a near universally attractive male form that tends to differ in size versus a vast difference in the proportions.

It is mainly a preference in the size of a mate vs. a completely different shift in body type preference. There is a reason that almost all main characters in romance novels have a similar description. Having a big, broad upper back and well-developed lats enhances the appearance of the shoulder-to-hip width ratio and really shows through when someone views you from the back. The reason why this is attractive is that men with greater upper body strength were on average more successful evolutionarily than ones without due to the challenges our ancestors faced and women evolved to find these cues attractive in their mates. Our psychology and preferences have not adjusted to our current lifestyle. This physique visually represents physical competence and strength in the upper body, which is one of the biggest differences amongst the sexes. So big of a difference in fact that many 13-year-old boys who have properly trained for just a short amount of time will be as strong as women who have been training their entire lives. Leg and lower body strength are very similar for both sexes when equated for size.

A proportionally larger and stronger upper body conveys strength and physical competence in men and men have a surprisingly significant amount of control over how their body is formed when it comes to building it the way they want to. If you are a thinner man, you are able to put on muscle in the right areas to create a dramatic shift in how your body appears if you work the right areas in the right ways. If you are a heavier person who tends to put on more fat, you can change your diet, do the right types of exercise to lose some of that fat, and put on muscle in specific areas to achieve an attractive physique. Some people are just born with a body type that is attractive to many women. Regardless of the genetic hand that you were dealt, you are able to change your circumstances.

While there are women who have physical type preferences that vary a bit, for instance, some may be particularly attracted to men with big arms, who are very lean, who have big shoulders, or big, ripped and vascular forearms, etc., we are going to focus on what is attractive to the most women.

When it comes to developing your body as a man, you will want to emphasize building big, broad, strong shoulders and a big, full chest as these are the primary physical attributes that are attractive to most women. (there have even been studies done that report that women who are with partners that are closest to the 1.62:1 shoulder to hip ratio tend to self-report having more orgasms than women who are with partners who aren't). When shown silhouettes of different male body types, women tend to consistently choose the same ones which as discussed earlier are pretty similar in general shape but differ in size, some choosing a lean Brad Pitt in Fight Club type physique and some choosing a Chris Hemsworth as Thor physique. This has also been shown to be irrespective of cultural influences as it is the case in many different countries with vastly different cultural influences and even in cultures that are essentially untouched by modern influences. You will also want to focus on building a big, broad upper back, traps, neck, and lats, as this will enhance the appearance of the v-shaped torso that women find attractive. Having a strong upper back and traps will give you a more aggressive, dominant appearance in the upper body and work to automatically place your shoulders into a strong, stable, pulled-back position that thrusts your chest out. In addition to the upper body, you will also want to develop a strong, powerful set of glutes, as they are essentially the seat of athleticism. The best athletes have strong, powerful hips that are capable of helping them sprint fast, jump high and far, throw knockout punches, hit bomb home runs, toss their opponents, and lift heavy shit. Almost every person, man or woman, can appreciate a nice ass.

This is because of the competence that is subconsciously conveyed through this feature (everything comes down to the competence that is subconsciously conveyed through the features, the features themselves are not inherently attractive). This is essentially the foundation, big strong, broad shoulders; a big, strong, full chest; big, broad, and strong upper back and lats; a thick neck and big traps (women actually pay attention to this area, which was surprising to me at first after hearing it first hand) and a big, strong and athletic set of glutes.

After you've put most of your emphasis into these areas, it's time to focus on the arms and forearms making them big, strong, and as vascular as possible. When it comes to legs, you will want them to be strong and lean but not necessarily big (think proportionate). When the legs get proportionately too big, they can make the body appear somewhat feminine as it increases the Appearance of a smaller waist-to-hip ratio, which is the foundation of attraction in women's bodies. This is not a reason to skip leg day but more so to emphasize strength, power, and leanness over pure size.

My theory about this is that when you build mass in the legs vs. building it in the hips/close to the hips such as the high hamstrings, the farther the center of mass in the legs is from the center of the body and the less efficient sprinting and running becomes in both endurance and speed and the ability to run long distances during a hunt is one of the main physical attributes that propelled the ascension of the human race to its throne as the uncontested apex predator of the planet. When you build a body that is inefficient at one or more of the primary reasons that fueled the ascension of your species, it is also unattractive (again, my theory), at least at a subconscious level.

It is important to remain proportionately built but typically, the women who find big legs and more specifically, the quads attractive are women who are into bodybuilding as the quads are a primary focus in bodybuilding competitions. If you want to enter into a bodybuilding competition or if your goal is ultimate strength, especially in the squat and/or sumo deadlift specifically, you'll need to emphasize building your quads but from an evolutionary attraction and athletic performance perspective, building this area up past a proportionate point can detract from your overall physique as a man. Women as something that catches their eye unless they look like they have never been trained before rarely mention calves. Any size that is put into the calves has the largest effect on bringing the center of mass of the legs farther away from the hips and thus has the largest detrimental impact on running efficiency and top-end speed. Some studies have even found that it is beneficial to have smaller calves/lower legs for sprinting as it is less mass for the hips and upper leg to move and is beneficial for speed/has a quicker turnover rate during sprinting. This is not to say do not train them but that they do not need to be a primary focus of your program if building the most attractive body possible is your goal. You should be training each part of your body at least a little bit so you can avoid having a weak link that results in an injury in or outside of the weight room.

When training the abs and torso, you will want to emphasize methods of training that create a lean and strong midsection. Having visible, lean, and cut abs is ideal while being shredded may be taking it a bit too far as this would appear on someone who was malnourished. The midsection is essentially the transmission of the body through which the power and strength generated in the upper and lower body is transferred and is a common area for injury as it's weak in many, if not most people. Strengthening your lower back, abs and oblique's will allow you to transfer the force generated through your legs and hips into your upper body more efficiently. This is important for many life activities and nearly all sports, as almost every sport requires this.

Hitting a golf ball, swinging a bat, throwing a fastball or passing a football, throwing a punch, throwing an opponent in wrestling/a fight/judo/etc., tackling an opponent, blocking someone, carrying groceries, carrying another person, shooting a gun and absorbing the recoil (becomes increasingly important the higher power and higher caliber the weapon is), squatting external weight and picking stuff up are all examples of why this is important in a real-world context. Because this area is prone to injury it is critical to build it with function being the primary intent while aesthetics should be secondary and will typically come as a byproduct of building it for function.

If your main goal with training is to build the most attractive, masculine body that you're capable of, focusing on a 3:2 ratio of upper-body to lower-body training sessions will likely get you there. If your primary goal is performance in a particular sport, you will have to adjust this ratio to accommodate the specific demands of your sport/activity.

One factor to consider as well is that many modern women, especially in Western or Westernized countries are on hormonal birth control which can affect their mate preferences causing them to be more attracted to men who are more feminine than they would otherwise be attracted to if their hormones weren't being altered by external factors. So the more masculine you are in appearance, mindset, personality, and actions, the more likely you will be attractive to feminine women in their hormonally unaltered state. A woman's hormonal cycle can also affect the type of men that she's attracted to, being more attracted to more masculine men when she's more fertile/ovulating and either having no change in preference or being attracted to less masculine men when she's not ovulating/less fertile (hence the shift in preference when taking hormonal birth control). Note:

Unrelated to fitness and performance, date your future wife/long-term partner while she's not on birth control to make sure she still finds you attractive and that you guys are a good long-term match! This is a personal theory of mine on why many of today's marriages are dissolving.

Women

While women tend to be generally attracted to a certain body type, men are a different story. There is a "market" per se of men for all shapes and sizes of women. There are groups of men who appreciate and are attracted to pretty much any shape and size of female body there is. While this is true, there are a few physical characteristics that many or even a majority of men are attracted to and you can really boil them down to physical indicators of health which will improve as you exercise, sleep better, eat cleaner and become overall healthier.

Clear, smooth, plump collagen-filled skin; long, lustrous, thick, and soft hair. A healthy amount of body fat is distributed to specific places (many men like women who are a bit softer and thicker than many women are tend to think). A bit of muscle, particularly in the legs and specifically in the glutes, low back and abs and some in the upper body, the broader the shoulders and more of a v-taper that a woman's body takes on, the more masculine of an appearance she will have. It's important to develop the area for functional purposes and make sure it's not neglected but not put the emphasis that a man would put into it if your goal is to develop your body in a way that's attractive to the largest pool of potential mates and aim to get as close to a .6-.7:1 waist to hip ratio (this waist to hip ratio has been shown to be a universal attraction cue as it is seen as attractive in nearly every culture regardless of media and various other cultural influences and has even been shown to be the case for almost any size woman).

When it comes to training frequency, somewhere around a 1-2:3 ratio of upper body to lower body training frequency with a specific focus on glute and posterior chain development seems to be effective when it comes to building an attractive, feminine body. Building an attractive body for a woman is simple when it comes down to it. Put your effort into getting healthy, building an ass (enhances the waist-to-hip ratio), eat in a way that supports some fat and a mostly soft but in shape body, but doesn't accumulate around the midsection (most men don't care if you have visible abs as long as you maintain the .6-.7:1 waist to hip ratio). Build a strong, tight, midsection including abs, oblique has and low back; and do some upper body training to build some but not a lot of muscle up there (essentially just enough to look like you do not neglect it but do not overemphasize it).

Of course, if you compete in a sport then your primary goal should be to functionally build your body to perform optimally for that sport but if you want to build your body in a way that will appear attractive to a large portion of the male population then it will help to put your effort into training in the ways discussed. In addition to the strength training and bodybuilding that you will be doing, you will want

To do some sort of aerobic exercise to improve blood flow and circulation throughout your body and to break a good, full-body sweat. The more the better as this will do wonders for your skin in keeping it clear, soft, smooth, and hydrated.

This is all it takes, it really is this simple. Just focus mostly on your lower body and core, do enough upper body to make sure you're staying proportional and that it looks like you don't neglect it and do enough cardio to keep your heart healthy, improve your circulation, and get a full-body sweat going (or use the sauna), you'll be in great shape! It is probably a lot less work than you imagine and you will feel great mentally afterwards.

Your mind will be in a much better place in regards to mood. You will improve the neuroplasticity of your brain making it easier to learn new stuff and in a way become smarter. You will be stronger and more physically independent, less likely to get sick, improve your bone density (important to start as early as possible and your younger years are critical for this but it is never too late (teens and twenties) and make yourself smoking hot to your current or future mate.

CHAPTER 4

Power

Power in human performance is essentially a type of strength and is your ability to generate a certain amount of force over a certain amount of time. Ultimately, every movement generates some degree of power but for the purposes of this book, we will be talking about high-power movement, generating as much force as possible over the shortest amount of time possible. These demonstrations could be in lifting a certain amount of weight fast, throwing an implement as far or as high as you can, jumping or sprinting. Once a base level of general strength is built, it is important to train for power as powerful movement is the basis for most sports and physical activity and as you age, is one of the first types of strength that you lose if you do not train for it. For this book, we are going to keep things relatively simple as training for this type of strength can potentially get complex.

This skill comes and goes relatively quickly so it is important to keep training for it consistently. It is also relatively specific, although there is some transference between movements so it is important to focus on the type of movements that you see yourself having to use in whatever sports or physical activities you are going to be participating in. It is my belief that you should be using all the different types of movements listed but you should emphasize the ones you will be using most. The most commonly used movement types are sprints, jumps, throws, Olympic lifts (snatches, cleans and jerks and all of their variants) and the powerlifts (bench press, squats, deadlifts) performed explosively using bands or chains

As a basis of your power training, it is easy and time-efficient to just rotate through the various types of movement each training session and to do them after you do a general warm-up. To start, you will want to start easing into it and increasing your level of effort as you get more warmed up and primed to go. Your training session for sprinting, jumping, or throwing could look something like this (after general warm-up): 1 effort at about 50% intensity, 1 effort at about 60%, 1 effort at about 70%, Then hit your working sets at around 80-90% effort for 3-5 sets, stopping either right after or just before you see a drop off in your performance. For lifting, you would use between 30% and 85% of your max in total resistance (utilizing bands and chains, if desired and available) performed with the intent to move the weight as fast as you're capable of for each rep and for the set as a whole performing 5-12 sets of 1-5 reps depending on the percentage of your 1 rep max that you choose to use. *You can utilize what is called Prilepin's Chart, essentially a chart/table that you can use as a guide to determine how many sets, reps, and the total volume of a movement you should perform in a workout to get an effective training stimulus at any given percentage. This chart can be found online by doing a quick Google search.

A standard structure for implementing this style of training could look like the following:

1. General warm-up and mobility

2. High Speed, Low Force Power Training - 3-5 sets of one of the following (for simplicity's sake)

   a. Throw

   b. Sprint

   c. Jump

3. Medium Speed, Medium Force Power Training - 5-12 sets of one or two of the following, each done as explosively as possible

   a. Power or Muscle Snatch

   b. Power or Muscle Clean

   c. Squat Variation using the Compensatory Acceleration method or Accommodating Resistance such as bands or chains

    d. Deadlift variation using the Compensatory Acceleration method or Accommodating Resistance such as bands or chains

    e. Bench Press variation using the Compensatory Acceleration method or Accommodating Resistance such as bands or chains

    f. Pull Up or Row variation using the Compensatory Acceleration method or Accommodating Resistance such as bands or chains

4. Movement Specific ROM Strength and Muscle Building Assistance Lift a. choose 1-2 lifts that strengthen the range of motion of a movement that you're weak in or that you fail the movement at

5. Muscle Building Assistance

    a. Choose 1-2 that target specific muscles that are underdeveloped

6. Core Exercise

    a. Use exercises to build the muscles of the lower back, abs and oblique's.

7. Durability Exercise

    a. Choose one exercise and perform 1-3 high rep sets to build an area that is particularly weak or injury prone for you.

CHAPTER 5

Durability

While strength training in general can be considered durability training, we will be focusing on utilizing high rep sets of banded exercises in particular (standard resistance also works but bands are more effective) to strengthen areas where the connective tissues are commonly prone to injury such as the hamstrings, adductors and triceps. Core/trunk/torso training will be included in this section as it has a particularly injury prone area in many people, especially people that do not know how to brace correctly during lifts (Valsalva maneuver). This section is fairly simple as you choose an area that feels particularly weak or that you may have injured before and do a bunch of reps at a fast and continuous pace of an exercise utilizing the stretch reflex as much as possible for its performance.

Using banded exercises seems to be particularly effective for these, as they tend to utilize the stored elastic energy of the tendons to a higher degree. (They are almost magical in this regard, if you ever have pain or soreness in what feels like the tendon area. The area that connects the muscle to the bone, do 100 reps as fast as you can of a banded isolation movement that targets those particular tendons, the next day, you'll almost certainly feel an improvement in how they feel).

The idea here is that you choose an isolation-type exercise and do 1-3 sets of 30-200 reps in a fast and continuous as possible way of a banded exercise that targets tendons that are achy or in an area that you may have injured before. It is that simple. It should feel like you have an extreme pump after doing this, as part of the reason that it is so effective is that it drives blood and nutrients to the area that is being worked. Tendons do not have an active blood supply and delivering the nutrients that repair and strengthen them is reliant on passive diffusion across the tissue.

You can do these as straight sets, you can pick out a number of reps you want to do and just get them done as quickly as you can taking as few breaks as possible for as short of a time as possible or just pick a band out and do as many reps as you possibly can as fast as you can for 1-3 sets. As long as you are doing these with the intent discussed, you do not need to put much thought into it as long as you are choosing the right muscles/tendons to target.

In terms of core training, you will want to train it in several different ways and from a variety of different angles. It is important to train it from all different sides, angles and directions in a controlled manner so when the inevitable accident occurs, it will be strong and resilient. The different types of core training you will want to focus on are flexion, extension, anti-extension, lateral flexion, anti-lateral extension, rotation and anti-rotation. You will want to focus on the primary types of loading that the core exhibits most in daily life, which are anti-flexion, anti-lateral flexion, anti-extension and anti-rotation keeping the body rigid the spine locked in place, which is the safest position for it. The "anti" aspect of the exercise generally just implies that it is a statically held position where you are resisting the type of movement that follows. The other methods of training are still important but the ones just referenced are the most important. Any exercise that trains these types of loading can be used, especially if it is relatively easy to increase the load of it so you can continually increase your strength in these positions.

Core/Trunk Exercises

Flexion - Weighted Sit-ups and Hanging Leg Raises

Anti-Flexion - Good mornings, Hip Extensions and Arch Holds

Extension - Super Mans, Back Extensions and Reverse Hypers

Anti-Extension - Ab Wheel and L-Sits

Lateral Flexion - Side Crunches and Oblique Crunches

Anti-Lateral Extension - Side Planks and Suitcase Carries

Rotation - Russian Twists and Banded Rotations

Anti-Rotation - All variations of Pall of Presses and Holds, Single Arm Kettlebell Swings, and Side Planks while performing a cable or band row

How to Put Everything Together

Now that you know how to apply all the different aspects of physical training and what each aspect does for you, the question is how you put all this together into an effective and efficient plan.

What you do and how much you do really depends on how much time you have to dedicate to your physical training and how creative you can get with your time efficiency (completing several things at once such as getting in your low intensity, restorative physical activity i.e. walking while also getting something else done such as meeting with a friend or business partner, listening to an audiobook or podcast, mentally rehearsing or visualizing a goal or business plan, etc.). If you have the time, are able to get creative and/or can make the time, the following is an optimal plan.

Weekly Goals

- 30+ minutes of low-intensity walking or hiking each day, ideally outside in nature but other low intensity physical activity will suffice. First thing in the morning is a great way to get your day started as exposing your eyes to sunlight as early as possible helps synchronize your circadian rhythm and is beneficial for your sleeping patterns. It also increases the production of BDNF in your brain, which is beneficial for learning and neuroplasticity. With this type of activity, the more, the better as longer durations increase BDNF to a higher degree. Working up to 8k-10k steps is a great ideal to shoot for throughout the whole day. This is a lot of easy physical activity but is closest to what our ancestors were doing daily just to acquire enough sustenance to live and thus what we have evolved to do. This takes a lot of time but if you can be efficient with it, you can combine this with several other activities and accomplish it. It definitely makes it easier when you make more active instead of sedentary choices.

- 2x per week do 30 minutes of moderate intensity cardio at a pace where you might be able to say a sentence but not talk continuously. This can be running, rowing, biking, fast hiking uphill, going on a fast walk with a weight vest on, sled dragging, etc.

- Strength, power, and hypertrophy training 4 days a week at a rate of 3 upper for every 2 lower body days for men and a rate of 2 upper body days for every 3 lower body days for women. Adding one bonus day that targets all the small, often neglected muscle groups missed during the rest of the week is also a good idea to avoid potential injuries due to undertrained areas.
  - If you noticed, the ratios listed do not add up to the 4 days a week, so some weeks you'll be performing more upper body days, and some weeks you'll be performing more lower body days. Just keep a constant rotation going and do four primary workouts plus the optional bonus workout.
- one time per week, perform some sort of high intensity sprint intervals on a bike, rower, pushing a prowler or sprinting uphill. The work effort should last 6-15 seconds with a 45-90 second active

Rest period for 6-15 total efforts performed at a near maximal intensity (think about as fast as you are able to go while maintaining your composure and technique). Start with the lowest amount of effort and increase over time. The rest period should last long enough that you can output the same intensity with each effort but no longer. Essentially the shortest possible time you need to take a break before being able to perform at the same level in each set. You should still be breathing heavily during these efforts but your muscles should be recovered.

How to Design Your Workouts

Men

For men, if your goal is aesthetics + performance (if it is pure performance or you have glaring weaknesses, you can restructure it to accommodate for those) the following structure for your weekly training should look like the following:

Day 1 - Upper Body Strength Focus

Note: 30 minute walk at some point during the day. Eightk+ steps ideal to shoot for throughout the day.

Resistance Workout

A - Pressing Strength Movement:

*Choose a bench press, overhead press, dip or push up variation. The goal is to perform the movement within the rep range that builds strength, 1-6 and work up to the heaviest weight you can do with your best technique.

B - Pulling Strength Movement:

*Choose a row, pulldown or pull up/chin up variation. The goal is to perform the movement within the rep range that builds strength, 1-6 and work up to the heaviest weight you can do with your best technique. When it comes to vertical pulling, if you are able to, alternating between pull ups/chin-ups and a pulldown variation works well. In terms of rowing variations, choosing the variation based on how fatigued your spinal muscles are and what you have planned for your lower body for the week works well. Opt for bent over barbell or Pendlay/Dead Stop rows if your spine is fresh and you do not have a heavy deadlift planned for later in the week. If you want to avoid loading your spine to a high degree inverted barbell, TRX or ring rows are a good option. Single arm dumbbell rows are also good for this purpose.

C - Chest Hypertrophy Movement:

*Choose an accessory exercise that builds the chest predominately. Dumbbell bench press/floor press, cable and dumbbell flyes (press + fly hybrids work really well for these), squeeze push-ups, and hex press all work well for these. Build it from all angles; especially incline variations and movements that target the upper chest.

D - Lateral Delt Hypertrophy Movement:

*Choose an accessory that builds the lateral delts specifically. Movements such as dumbbell lateral delt raises, cable lateral delt raises, incline bench side lying cross body lateral raises, leaning cross body lateral raises, face pull variations and weighted pass-through are all great options.

E - Upper Back/Lat Hypertrophy Movement:

*Choose an exercise that builds the muscles in the upper back and lats mainly. Typically, for this movement since you have already performed a pulling movement earlier in the workout, it is a

Good idea to choose something that can be performed for a bit higher reps (7-12 per set) and really targets the part of the back that is lagging the most for you. Since the lats are notoriously one of the most challenging places to "activate" or feel working, they are a lagging area for many people.

Day 2 - Lower Body Strength Focus

Note: 30 minute walk at some point during the day. 18k+ steps ideal to shoot for throughout the day.

Resistance Workout

A - Lower Strength Movement:

*Choose a deadlift, squat, good morning or lunge variation and work up to a technically sound 1-6 RM on it. It works well to rotate these from week to week or to

spend just 2-3 weeks working on a particular type of movement before rotating it to something else to avoid accommodation. B - Lower Strength Assistance Lift:

*Choose something that specifically builds a type of weakness you have, either builds a specific range of motion that you are weak in or builds a lagging muscle group. This could be one of the following (don't limit yourself to these but use them as ideas): Tempo Romanian Deadlifts if you're weak through the middle range on your deads, dimel deadlifts if you're weak at the top or deficit deadlifts just to your knees if you're weak from the floor on your pull. If you are weak in the bottom of a squat, you could do paused squats, pin squats or box squats from the height that you are weakest in. If it is, the middle range of motion that you are weakest in, you could pulse squats through just that range of motion where you do not go fully down or fully up and just work the middle range or if you are weak at the top of the squat, you could use bands or chains to strengthen that position.

C - Glute/Hip and Lower Back Accessory Movement:

*Choose a movement that builds the glutes, lower back and/or hamstrings. This movement is meant to be a more general-purpose low back, glute and hamstring strengthener and builder. Great choices for these would be hip extensions/back raises on the GHD machine or 45 degree back extension machine (banded, holding dumbbells or weight plate, deadlift style, etc.), reverse hypers (strict, standard, banded, etc.), Russian kettlebell swings,

D - Hamstring Accessory:

*Choose an isolation type movement that directly targets the hamstrings. Seated leg curls, standing leg curls, lying leg curls, GH raises and inverse leg curls are all good options. E - Core/Trunk Durability Accessory:

*Choose an exercise that strengthens your trunk in a way that you are weak in or that you need to be strong in for a sport you do. Choose a type of movement from the core/trunk exercises mentioned earlier in the book and do 3-5 challenging sets of them.

Day 3 - Restoration and Aerobic Training

Note: 30 minute walk at some point during the day. 8k+ steps ideal to shoot for throughout the day.

Aerobic Training: 30-45 minutes at pace you can talk a sentence possibly but not have a continuous conversation at.

Optional Resistance Training for Calves and Tibialis

Day 4 - Upper Body Speed/Hypertrophy Focus

Note: 30 minute walk at some point during the day. 8k+ steps ideal to shoot for throughout the day.

Resistance Workout

A - Pressing Hypertrophy or Speed Movement:

*Choose a bench press, overhead press, dip or push up variation and perform it at 65-85% of one RM with the intent to move the weight as fast as possible or to move it for as many reps as you are able to do. When performing speed work, you will want to do 4-12 sets of 2-5 reps, essentially staying in a rep range that allows all reps to be performed with the same high quality speed. Search for Prilepin's chart on google and use it to determine the number of sets and reps you should do at any given percentage. If you choose to work hypertrophy on these, perform the movements with a fast or explosive concentric, a slow eccentric and possibly a pause at the bottom of the movement where they muscles you are working are under the most stretch. It works well to work on one goal (speed or hypertrophy) for 6-9 weeks at a time then switch to the other for a similar amount of time.

B - Pulling Hypertrophy or Speed Movement:

*Choose a row, pulldown or pull up/chin up variation and perform it at 65-85% of one RM with the intent to move the weight as fast as possible or to move it for as many reps as you are able to do. Search for Prilepin's chart on google and use it to determine the number of sets and reps you should do at any given percentage.

Typically, hypertrophy style movements work really well for this area interspersed with periods of power/speed training. When it comes to vertical pulling, if you are able to, alternating between pull-ups/chin-ups and a pulldown variation works well. In terms of rowing variations, choosing the variation based on how fatigued your spinal muscles are and what you have planned for your lower body for the week works well. Opt for bent over barbell or Pendlay/Dead Stop rows if your spine is fresh and you do not have a heavy deadlift planned for later in the week. If you want to avoid loading your spine to a high degree inverted barbell, TRX or ring rows are a good option. Single arm dumbbell rows are also good for this purpose.

C - Chest Hypertrophy Movement:

*Choose an accessory exercise that builds the chest predominantly. Dumbbell bench press/floor press, cable and dumbbell flyes (press + fly hybrids work really well for these), squeeze push-ups, and hex press all work well for these. Build it from all angles; especially incline variations and movements that target the upper chest.

D - Lateral Delt Hypertrophy Movement:

*Choose an accessory that builds the lateral delts specifically. Movements such as dumbbell lateral delt raises, cable lateral delt raises, incline bench side lying cross body lateral raises, leaning cross body lateral raises, face pull variations and weighted pass-through are all great options.

E - Upper Back/Lat Hypertrophy Movement:

*Choose an exercise that builds the muscles in the upper back and lats mainly. Typically, for this movement since you have already performed a pulling movement earlier in the workout, it is a

A good idea to choose something that can be performed for a bit higher reps (7-12 per set) and really targets the part of the back that is lagging the most for you. Since the lats are notoriously one of the most challenging places to "activate" or feel working, they are a lagging area for many people.

Day 5 - Lower Body Speed/Hypertrophy Focus

Note: 30 minute walk at some point during the day. 8k+ steps ideal to shoot for throughout the day.

Resistance Workout

A - Lower Strength Movement:

*Choose a deadlift, squat, good morning or lunge variation and perform it at 65-85% of one RM with the intent to move the weight as fast as possible or to move it for as many reps as you are able to do. When performing

speed work, you will want to do 4-12 sets of 2-5 reps, essentially staying in

A rep range that allows all reps to be performed with the same high quality speed. Search for Prilepin's chart on google and use it to determine the number of sets and reps you should do at any given percentage. If you choose to work hypertrophy on this movement, perform the movement with a fast or explosive concentric, a slow eccentric and possibly a pause at the bottom of the movement where they muscles you are working are under the most stretch. It works well to work on one goal (speed or hypertrophy) for 6-9 weeks at a time then switch to the other for a similar amount of time.

B - Lower Strength Assistance Lift:

*Choose something that specifically builds a type of weakness you have, either builds a specific range of motion that you are weak in or builds a lagging muscle group. This could be one of the following (don't limit yourself to these but use them as ideas): Tempo Romanian Deadlifts if you're weak through the middle range on your deads, dimel deadlifts if you're weak at the top or deficit deadlifts just to your knees if you're weak from the floor on your pull. If you are weak in the bottom of a squat, you could do paused squats, pin squats or box squats from the height that you are weakest in. If it is, the middle range of motion that you are weakest in, you could pulse squats through just that range of motion

where you do not go fully down or fully up and just work the middle range or if you are weak at the top of the squat, you could use bands or chains to strengthen that position.

C - Glute/Hip and Lower Back Accessory Movement:

*Choose a movement that builds the glutes, lower back and/or hamstrings. This movement is meant to be a more general-purpose low back, glute and hamstring strengthener and builder. Great choices for these would be hip extensions/back raises on the GHD machine or 45 degree back extension machine (banded, holding dumbbells or weight plate, deadlift style, etc.), reverse hypers (strict, standard, banded, etc.), Russian kettlebell swings,

D - Hamstring Accessory:

*Choose an isolation type movement that directly targets the hamstrings. Seated leg curls, standing leg curls, lying leg curls, GH raises and inverse leg curls are all good options. E - Core/Trunk Durability Accessory:

*Choose an exercise that strengthens your trunk in a way that you are weak in or that you need to be strong in for a sport you do. Choose a type of movement from the core/trunk exercises mentioned earlier in the book and do 3-5 challenging sets of them.

Day 6 - Low Volume Upper Accessory or Hybrid Upper + Lower and HIIT

Note: 30 minute walk at some point during the day. 8k+ steps ideal to shoot for throughout the day.

Low Volume Resistance Workout

*2-3 sets of each exercise depending on how fatigued and sore the body is feeling (opt for two sets most of the time). Higher reps, 8+ each set. The goal of this day is to do exercises that feel great for the areas and get a good pump/blood flow going to them. No movements that feel like an excessive amount of strain to the connective tissues is occurring. This can consist of all banded work if you want to or need to improve the durability of the areas you work or your body is feeling achy.

A - Small/Isolation Chest Hypertrophy Exercise:

*Choose an isolation type movement that works the pecs such as cable or band flyes, dumbbell flyes, etc. Lighter calisthenics such as push-ups and dips work well for this part of the program as well. Perform with a slow negative/eccentric, a fast concentric and a 1-3 second pause at the point of the most stretch.

B - Lateral Delt Isolation Hypertrophy Exercise:

*Choose an isolation style exercise that preferentially works the lateral delts such as dumbbell lateral delt raises, cable lateral delt raises, incline bench side lying cross body lateral raises, leaning cross body lateral raises, face pull variations and weighted pass-through (these are a great full spectrum shoulder developing exercise if you have the tools to do them and your shoulders tolerate them well) Perform with a slow negative/eccentric, a fast concentric and a 1-3 second pause at the point of the most stretch.

C - Upper Back/Lat Hypertrophy Exercise:

*Choose an exercise that works the lats and upper back but does not load the spine (no unsupported barbell or dumbbell rows, chest supported rows are OK). These can be higher rep pull-ups or chin-ups; a pulldown (unilateral or bilateral) variation; inverted barbell rows, TRX rows or ring rows; or a chest supported row variation. Perform with a slow negative/eccentric, a fast concentric and a 1-3 second pause at the point of the most stretch.

D - Biceps Isolation Hypertrophy Exercise:

*Choose an exercise that targets the biceps such as hammer curls, cable curls, standard dumbbell curls, band curls, etc. Perform with a slow negative/eccentric and a fast concentric. E - Triceps Isolation Hypertrophy Exercise:

*Choose an exercise that targets the triceps such as rope or band press downs, v bar press downs, Tate Presses, dumbbell rollback extensions, etc. Perform with a slow negative/eccentric and a fast concentric.

F - Rear Delt Isolation Hypertrophy Exercise:

*Choose an exercise that targets the rear delts such as rear delt raises, side lying rear delt raises, cable or band face pulls, elbows out ring or cable cross rows, upright rows or band pull aparts. Perform with a slow negative/eccentric and a fast concentric.

Optional: Add in a couple sets of calf training exercise, Tibialis training exercises, lower intensity hamstring isolation exercises and/or a couple sets of higher rep back extensions or reverse hypers if your lower body is lagging a bit.

HIIT/Sprints

Perform 5-15 short duration (6-15 seconds), high intensity sprints on a low impact aerobics machine such as a rower, ski erg, spin bike or ideally, an air bike with both upper and lower body components like the Assault bike. Rest should be long enough to maintain intensity but not long enough to fully slow down breathing (recover to around 60% of MHR and go again), usually around 1-2 minutes.

Day 7 - Rest, Recovery and Restoration

Note: 30-60 minute walk or restorative yoga at some point during the day. Utilize contrast/hot-cold therapy, sauna, hot tub, massage/body work, etc. if the body is feeling particularly sore or achy.

Women

For women, if your goal is aesthetics + performance (if it is pure performance or you have glaring weaknesses, you can restructure it to accommodate for those) the following structure for your weekly training should look like the following:

Day 1 - Lower Body Strength Focus

Note: 30 minute walk at some point during the day. 8k steps over the course of the day is ideal.

Resistance Workout

A - Lower Strength Movement:

*Choose a glute focused deadlift, squat, good morning or lunge variation and work up to a technically sound 1-6 RM on it. It works well to rotate these from week to week or to spend just 2- 3 weeks working on a particular type of movement before rotating it to something else to avoid accommodation. Choose movements you have good mind-muscle connection to in the glutes and utilize proper cueing to increase recruitment in that region.

B - Lower Strength Assistance Lift:

*Choose something that specifically builds a type of weakness you have, either builds a specific range of motion that you are weak in or builds a lagging muscle group. This could be one of the following (don't limit yourself to these but use them as ideas): Tempo Romanian Deadlifts if you're weak through the middle range on your deads, dimel deadlifts if you're weak at the top or deficit deadlifts just to your knees if you're weak from the floor on your pull. If you are weak in the bottom of a squat, you could do paused squats, pin squats or box squats from the height that you are weakest in. If it is, the middle range of motion that you are weakest in, you could pulse squats through just that range of motion where you do not go fully down or fully up and just work the middle range or if you are weak at the top of the squat, you could use bands or chains to strengthen that position. For aesthetic purposes choose movements that do these things and recruit the glutes to a high degree.

C - Glute/Hip and Lower Back Accessory Movement:

*Choose a movement that builds the glutes, lower back and/or hamstrings. This movement is meant to be a more general-purpose low back, glute and hamstring strengthener and builder. Great choices for these would be hip extensions/back raises on the GHD machine or 45 degree back extension machine (banded, holding dumbbells or weight plate, deadlift style, etc.), reverse hypers (strict, standard, banded, etc.), Russian kettlebell swings,

D - Hamstring Accessory:

*Choose an isolation type movement that directly targets the hamstrings. Seated leg curls, standing leg curls, lying leg curls, GH raises and inverse leg curls are all good options. E - Core/Trunk Durability Accessory:

*Choose an exercise that strengthens your trunk in a way that you are weak in or that you need to be strong in for a sport you do. Choose a type of movement from the core/trunk exercises mentioned earlier in the book and do 3-5 challenging sets of them.

Day 2 - Upper Body Strength Focus

Note: 30 minute walk at some point during the day. 8k steps is ideal.

Resistance Workout

A - Pressing Strength Movement:

*Choose a bench press, overhead press, dip or push up variation. The goal is to perform the movement within the rep range that builds strength, 1-6 and work up to the heaviest weight you can do with your best technique.

B - Pulling Strength Movement:

*Choose a row, pulldown or pull up/chin up variation. The goal is to perform the movement within the rep range that builds strength, 1-6 and work up to the heaviest weight you can do with your best technique. When it comes to vertical pulling, if you are able to, alternating between pull ups/chin-ups and a pulldown variation works well. In terms of rowing variations, choosing the variation based on how fatigued your spinal muscles are and what you have planned for your lower body for the week works well. Opt for bent over barbell or Pendlay/Dead Stop rows if your spine is fresh and you do not have a heavy deadlift planned for later in the week. If you want to avoid loading your spine to a high degree inverted barbell, TRX or ring rows are a good option. Single arm dumbbell rows are also good for this purpose.

C - Chest Hypertrophy Movement:

*Choose an accessory exercise that builds the chest predominately. Dumbbell bench press/floor press, cable and dumbbell flyes (press + fly hybrids work really well for these), squeeze push-ups, and hex press all work well for these. Build it from all angles; especially incline variations and movements that target the upper chest.

D - Lateral Delt Hypertrophy Movement:

*Choose an accessory that builds the lateral delts specifically. Movements such as dumbbell lateral delt raises, cable lateral delt raises, incline bench side lying cross body lateral raises, leaning cross body lateral raises, face pull variations and weighted pass-through are all great options.

E - Upper Back/Lat Hypertrophy Movement:

*Choose an exercise that builds the muscles in the upper back and lats mainly. Typically, for this movement since you have already performed a pulling movement earlier in the workout, it is a good idea to choose something that can be performed for a bit higher reps (7-12 per set) and really targets the part of the back that is lagging the most for you. Since the lats are notoriously one of the most challenging places to "activate" or feel working, they are a lagging area for many people.

Day 3 - Restoration and Aerobic Training

Note: 30 minute walk at some point during the day. 8k steps is ideal.

Aerobic Training: 30-45 minutes at pace you can talk a sentence possibly but not have a continuous conversation at.

Optional Resistance Training for Calves and Tibialis

Day 4 - Lower Body Speed/Hypertrophy Focus

Note: 30 minute walk at some point during the day. 8k steps is ideal.

Resistance Workout

A - Lower Strength Movement:

*Choose a glute focused deadlift, squat, good morning or lunge variation and perform it at 65- 85% of 1 RM with the intent to move the weight as fast as possible or to move it for as many reps as you are able to do. When performing speed work, you will want to do 4-12 sets of 2-5 reps, essentially staying in a rep range that allows all reps to be performed with the same high quality speed. Search for Prilepin's chart on google and use it to determine the number of sets and reps you should do at any given percentage. If you choose to work hypertrophy on this movement, perform the movement with a fast or explosive concentric, a slow eccentric and possibly a pause at the bottom of the movement where the muscles you are working are under the most stretch. It works well to work on one goal (speed or hypertrophy) for 6-9 weeks at a time then switch to the other for a similar amount of time.

B - Lower Strength Assistance Lift:

*Choose something that specifically builds a type of weakness you have, either builds a specific range of motion that you are weak in or builds a lagging muscle group. This could be one of the following (don't limit yourself to these but use them as ideas): Tempo Romanian Deadlifts if you're weak through the middle range on your deads, dimel deadlifts if you're weak at the top or deficit deadlifts just to your knees if you're weak from the floor on your pull. If you are weak in the bottom of a squat, you could do paused squats, pin squats or box squats from the height that you are weakest in. If it is, the middle range of motion that you are weakest in, you could pulse squats through just that range of motion where you do not go fully down or fully up and just work the middle range or if you are weak at the top of the squat, you could use bands or chains to strengthen that position. If aesthetics are your goal, choose exercises for this part of the program that you feel predominantly in the glutes and that are known to be good glute builders. C - Glute/Hip and Lower Back Accessory Movement:

*Choose a movement that builds the glutes, lower back and/or hamstrings. This movement is meant to be a more general-purpose low back, glute and hamstring strengthener and builder. Great choices for these would be hip extensions/back raises on the GHD machine or 45 degree back extension machine (banded, holding dumbbells or weight plate, deadlift style, etc.), reverse hypers (strict, standard, banded, etc.), Russian kettlebell swings,

D - Hamstring Accessory:

*Choose an isolation type movement that directly targets the hamstrings. Seated leg curls, standing leg curls,

lying leg curls, GH raises and inverse leg curls are all good options. E - Core/Trunk Durability Accessory:

*Choose an exercise that strengthens your trunk in a way that you are weak in or that you need to be strong in for a sport you do. Choose a type of movement from the core/trunk exercises mentioned earlier in the book and do 3-5 challenging sets of them.

Day 5 - Upper Body Speed/Hypertrophy Focus

Note: 30 minute walk at some point during the day. 8k steps is ideal.

Resistance Workout

A - Pressing Hypertrophy or Speed Movement:

*Choose a bench press, overhead press, dip or push up variation and perform it at 65-85% of one RM with the intent to move the weight as fast as possible or to move it for as many reps as you are able to do. When performing speed work, you will want to do 4-12 sets of 2-5 reps, essentially staying in a rep range that allows all reps to be performed with the same high quality speed. Search for Prilepin's chart on google and use it to determine the number of sets and reps you should do at any given percentage. If you choose to work hypertrophy on these, perform the movements with a fast or explosive concentric, a slow eccentric and possibly a pause at the bottom of the movement where the muscles you are working are under the most stretch. It works well to work on one goal (speed or hypertrophy) for 6-9 weeks at a time then switch to the other for a similar amount of time.

B - Pulling Hypertrophy or Speed Movement:

*Choose a row, pulldown or pull up/chin up variation and perform it at 65-85% of one RM with the intent to move the weight as fast as possible or to move it for as many reps as you are able to do. Search for Prilepin's chart on google and use it to determine the number of sets and reps you should do at any given percentage. Typically, hypertrophy style movements work really well for this area interspersed with periods of power/speed training. When it comes to vertical pulling, if you are able to, alternating between pull-ups/chin-ups and a pulldown variation works well. In terms of rowing variations, choosing the variation based on how fatigued your spinal muscles are and what you have planned for your lower body for the week works well. Opt for bent over barbell or Pendlay/Dead Stop rows if your spine is fresh and you do not have a heavy deadlift planned for later in the week. If you want to avoid loading your spine to a high degree inverted barbell, TRX or ring rows are a good option. Single arm dumbbell rows are also good for this purpose.

C - Chest Hypertrophy Movement:

*Choose an accessory exercise that builds the chest predominantly. Dumbbell bench press/floor press, cable and dumbbell flyes (press + fly hybrids work really well for these), squeeze push-ups, and hex press all work well for these. Build it from all angles; especially incline variations and movements that target the upper chest.

D - Lateral Delt Hypertrophy Movement:

*Choose an accessory that builds the lateral delts specifically. Movements such as dumbbell lateral delt raises, cable lateral delt raises, incline bench side lying cross body lateral raises, leaning cross body lateral raises, face pull variations and weighted pass-through are all great options.

E - Upper Back/Lat Hypertrophy Movement:

*Choose an exercise that builds the muscles in the upper back and lats mainly. Typically, for this movement since you have already performed a pulling movement earlier in the workout, it is a good idea to choose something that can be performed for a bit higher reps (7-12 per set) and really targets the part of the back that is lagging the most for you. Since the lats are notoriously one of the most challenging places to "activate" or feel working, they are a lagging area for many people.

Day 6 - Low Volume Posterior Chain, Glute Isolation and HIIT

Note: 30 minute walk at some point during the day. 8k steps is ideal.

Low Volume Resistance Workout

*2-3 sets of each exercise depending on how fatigued and sore the body is feeling (opt for two sets most of the time). Higher reps, 8+ each set. The goal of this day is to do exercises that feel great for the areas and get a good pump/blood flow going to them. No movements that feel like an excessive amount of strain to the connective tissues is occurring. This can consist of all banded work if you want to or need to improve the durability of the areas you work or your body is feeling achy.

A - Full Glute Dominant Exercise:

*Choose an exercise that works the full gluteal region (upper and lower) such as Russian kettlebell swings, hip extensions on the GHD or 45 degree hyperextension machine (single leg is ideal but bilateral is also good), reverse hypers (strict, banded, unilateral or bilateral), kickbacks and glute bridges/hip thrusts (especially deficit to increase range of motion).

B - Secondary Glute Dominant Exercise:

*Choose a second exercise that works the full gluteal region (upper and lower) such as Russian kettlebell swings, hip extensions on the GHD or 45 degree hyper-extension machine (single leg is ideal but bilateral is also good), reverse hypers (strict, banded, unilateral or bilateral), kickbacks and glute bridges/hip thrusts (especially deficit to increase range of motion). If you choose hip extensions for exercise A, a good secondary choice would be reverse hypers to work the glutes from the other end of the body. Forward sled drags with the straps of the sled attached to a weight belt around your waist are an excellent way to target the glutes, hips and hamstrings in a low risk way and should be done regularly for this part of the program if you have access to a sled and a place to use it.

C - Side Glute Dominant Exercise:

*Choose exercises that build the sides of the glutes such as side plank clamshells, lateral sled walks, monster walks, etc.

D - Low Intensity Hamstring Isolation and Hypertrophy Exercise:

*Since ACL problems are more common in women due to biomechanical differences in men's and women's hips, and hamstring strengthening can prevent ACL injuries, it's important to regularly perform exercises that strengthen and build that area of the body. For this day, since you have already performed higher intensity hamstring strengthening exercises, choose something that still hits the spot but is not a "big" movement. These can be any type of machine leg curl such as a seated, standing or lying leg curl using a machine or bands.

HIIT/Sprints

Perform 5-15 short duration (6-15 second), high intensity sprints on a low impact aerobics machine such as a rower, ski erg, spin bike or ideally, an air bike with both upper and lower body components like the Assault bike. Rest should be long enough to maintain intensity but not long enough to fully slow down breathing (recover to around 60% of MHR and go again), usually around 1-2 minutes.

Day 7 - Rest, Recovery and Restoration

Note: 30-60 minute walk or restorative yoga at some point during the day. Utilize contrast/hot-cold therapy, sauna, hot tub, massage/body work, etc. if the body is feeling particularly sore or achy.

Conclusion

Now that you have the tools to take your health, physique, strength and fitness to optimal levels, it is up to you to put it to use. This is a more or less optimal blueprint of how to achieve peak health, fitness and aesthetics and if all the tools are utilized there can be a significant time cost but that time cost will be made up for in the health benefits you receive. I believe that it is important to know what is optimal so you can gauge where you are at accurately and decide what you have the time to dedicate to each day and how you can be efficient with your time. If you get the other aspects of your life in order such as your sleep, stress and diet and you put all of what is contained within these chapters to use, you will be in the best shape of your life aesthetically, health wise and in your performance.

Every part of this plan has a place and a different effect on your body, mind, and well-being. Strength training helps you become more physically competent, capable and independent, improving your confidence in life and helps your body prevent disease as the nutrients you consume will go towards building, repairing and powering muscle and activity instead of being stored as fat which can accumulate around the organs in an unhealthy way. Aerobic training affects your general well-being, your mood, your health, your mind and your nervous system in many ways, balancing it out and regulating it. Increasing your physical activity promotes learning, cognition and intelligence by creating the optimal environment in your body and mind to facilitate learning and memory through the increased blood flow and production of different factors and hormones in your body such as BDNF.

When it comes to optimal health, performance and aesthetics, taking a multifaceted approach to your training is the way to go as each part contributes something different to the unified whole of fitness and health.